Dr. Ben's
Bogus Diet
BREAKTHROUGH

The diet and exercise
revolution for people who
are definitely not serious

Ben Goode

The Truth About Life™

Published by:
Apricot Press
Box 1611
American Fork, Utah
84003

books @apricotpress.com
www.apricotpress.com

ISBN 1-885027-32-X

Cover Design & Layout by David Mecham
Printed in the United States of America

Our Guarantee

WE GUARANTEE THAT: Not following through on Dr. Ben's Bogus Diet and Exercise Breakthrough will get you pretty much the same results as not following through on some pretty famous and expensive diet and exercise programs. Plus, with this particular diet, you get the added benefit of being guilt-free because nobody expects you to succeed at this one. That's right. There are absolutely no guarantees here; we promise. When you fail at Dr. Ben's Bogus Diet Breakthrough that's exactly what's expected, because you know going in, that this one is pretty much just a bunch of hooey. You don't expect to lose any actual weight, get buns of steel or abs of iron. You can even keep your chins of cellulite if you want. We're perfectly OK with that.

Another great benefit with this book is that if you really think about it you realize that, whenever you do some other diet and exercise program you're wasting perfectly good calories and food by just burning them up for no good reason on the treadmill, track or bicycle. With our program, you don't necessarily have to waste even one calorie if you don't want to. You can use and enjoy 'em all! Good luck!

Ben Goode

- PART 1 -

- PART II -

Introduction

This book is written in two parts. The first part is for people who know darned good and well that they aren't going to really do anything serious about getting in shape and losing weight, yet making some kind of commitment to their health and well being makes them feel good. Many of these people also want everyone else to think they're trendy and are doing something about their weight and health and to have something in common with some of the other more self-disciplined people they hang out with.

The second part of the book is for those who sincerely believe that by some miracle, this time they are REALLY going to do it; that finally modern science has discovered the diet and exercise plan, which defies human nature and will actually work for them. Now is their moment of triumph. (All their friends are of course awaiting another good laugh at their expense and one of them is going to make a pile of money by being the one to get the closest to guessing the exact day and time when the dieter blows it again.) Part two was written to be a gift given by these friends as their contribution to the futile effort. It will also give them something productive to do besides just winking at one another.

HOW TO PROCEED

We have produced this potentially Pulitzer Prize-winning book because we know that for generations-ever since being chubby was considered cool, these two large groups have been literarily disenfranchised in our society. As far as we know, with the exception of this book, all diet and exercise books have been written exclusively for people who actually wanted a diet and exercise program, thereby leaving out over half the population by my estimates. That means, up until now, millions, even billions of people had absolutely no place to spend their money when what they needed was a trendy fad diet and exercise program so they could consider themselves "with it", but they didn't necessarily want to actually do any dieting or exercising. So, I guess, in that sense you could probably consider this a humanitarian gesture, too, which actually should get us into the Nobel Prize category and hopefully some extra publicity and sales.

DR. BEN'S BOGUS DIET BREAKTHROUGH

- PART ONE -

1 DR. BEN'S BOGUS SECRETS

Some of you may ask, "Why another diet book? There are millions, possibly billions of diet books and exercise programs out there already, and surely ONE of them ought to do the job." The truth is we have no idea about that. There very well could already be at least one diet and exercise book on the market that works for somebody, maybe even you. If that book should surface, we're just fine with that. In fact, since some of you may be worried about this, we'll put you right on the path to health and good looks before we actually even get into our book. In fact, without even looking through any of the competition's books, we can tell you the secret to looking and feeling great. Let's do that right now so we can get it out of the way early.

THE NUMBER ONE SECRET TO HEALTH, FITNESS, AND AN ATTRACTIVE YOU (drum roll please...)

The number one secret to diet and exercise success is to be born with a naturally high metabolism, solid muscle mass, and long legs. Somehow you need to manage this hereditary metabolism, long legs, and muscle mass stuff; otherwise, everything else is pretty much a waste of time.

We know this probably comes as no great surprise to those of you with low metabolisms and short legs who have tried everything from grapefruit rinds to Himalayan triathlons, but thinking about it can be kind of discouraging. So let's not dwell on it any longer. Sorry for bringing up such a painful subject.

Since we're admitting the truth up front, it should be obvious early on that we aren't trying to sell you another diet and exercise book that claims it will actually change your life. Just like you, we can't bear the thought of setting ourselves up for another failure. So, the heck with that. Our purpose with the Dr. Ben's Bogus diet is to achieve fad status so we can make millions of dollars quickly before everything in our diet is proven to kill you. This financial freedom strategy has proven highly successful for millions of snake-oil entrepreneurs in the past.

So, if you're the kind of person who has tried all those other diets before and failed or succeeded for a short time and then ballooned to twice your previous weight, if you are the type of person who likes his or her food, who knows that if you start another diet, you will just blow it again anyway, and who, knowing all that, wants to hang onto some self esteem and feel like you are doing something, however futile, for your own health, appearance and well being, this book is for you.

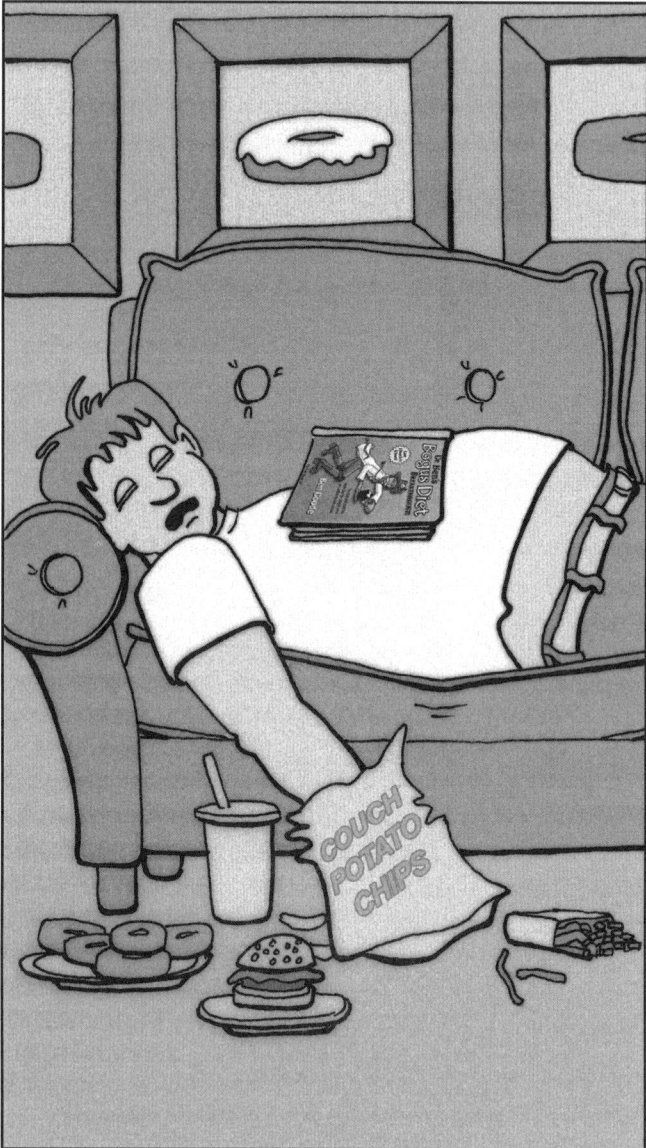

2 THE PARTICULARS OF DR. BEN'S BOGUS DIET AND EXERCISE PROGRAM

Here's the deal: You know perfectly well that with your attitude, you probably have a better chance of single-handedly conquering all the stupidity in the world or of curing the incompetent drivers on the road, than you do of really becoming fit and healthy.

So it also follows that, you probably also stand a better chance of changing the world's popular perception of chubby unathletic people than you do of actually becoming fit and healthy yourself, so with the Dr. Ben's Bogus Diet Breakthrough, I say we concentrate on the areas where we have the greatest potential for success, and since I'm the one writing the book, naturally I get what I want.

You already know that there are some things you simply are not going to do. For example, you know you should exercise regularly. Every cretin on the planet knows that. You've started over a million times and you've cheated and then petered out a million times more. And so if you get yourself all psyched up to go out there and try again you know that's what's likely to happen. So why beat yourself up about it. Face reality. The healthy you with the great body ain't gonna happen. Dr. Ben is OK with that.

You know perfectly well you should change what you eat. Every Bozo on the planet knows he should eat healthy. You've committed to change a million times and you've cheated your way out of the commitment a million times. Time to face reality. It ain't gonna happen. In the past, you couldn't even stick to a fad diet long enough to get sick so you could get in on the class action lawsuits that came later. So lets focus on the things that you **WILL** do. You might as well get some credit for that, don't you think?

TWO THINGS YOU WILL DO

#1 You **WILL** eat the stuff you like, even sneak it and then lie about it. So let's definitely put that down. You **WILL** eat pizza, pasta, carbs of all kinds, hamburgers, Mexican food, desserts and fully-sugared soda.

#2 You **WILL** also worry about dying from a stroke or heart attack or cancer; you **WILL** worry about your weight, how you look, and your overall health, at least when you start to lose it, so let's put that down too.

6

It stands to reason that in order to give you the greatest chance for diet and exercise success, we need to make these two principles the under girding theme of our diet and exercise program.

THE TWO MAIN PRINCIPLES OF DR. BEN'S BOGUS DIET AND EXERCISE PROGRAM

Principle #1 Eat Whatever You Want
Principle #2 Worry About it

For the first time in your life, you, my diet and exercise person, are finally standing on the threshold of diet and exercise success. You have a revolutionary program at which even YOU can succeed. Imagine how great you will feel having finally made a diet and exercise program actually work for you. Imagine how wonderful we will feel knowing that we made your success possible and got rich in the process.

CHANGING THE WORLD'S PERCEPTION

When it comes to diet and exercise programs, one other thing we have on our side is the fact that obesity is the number one health problem in the U.S. and most of the world, and it's only getting worse. So you know there are lots more people like you than there are skinny, fit ones. While we're at it, why don't we use that numerical advantage to change the world's perception of the rest of us? Obesity is a disease. I caught mine stomping through the jungles of Wendy's.

Think about it. Millions and billions of people out there are not fit and healthy. They have no representation. Changing the world's perception of people who don't take care of themselves sounds to me like a great and honorable undertaking, much more needed than coming up with the ten millionth strategy for futilely trying to lose weight.

So, instead of committing to a diet and exercise program that we know perfectly well we won't stick to, instead, let's use our energy to change everyone else's perceptions about being unfit and unhealthy. This is a terrific public service that will help millions and billions of people.

HOW TO CHANGE THE WORLD'S PERCEPTION AND MAKE BEING UNFIT TRENDY AGAIN

We have no idea. Let's just say that topic is outside the purview of this particular book, which will give us a good reason to follow it up with another one.

Now, with that out of the way, let me give you a few great tips that can really help you stick to Dr. Ben's diet and exercise program.

A COMPREHENSIVE LIST OF GREAT-TASTING FOODS THAT ARE ALSO GOOD FOR YOU

1.

A COMPREHENSIVE LIST OF FOODS THAT WON'T KILL YOU

1. Tofu
2. Broccoli

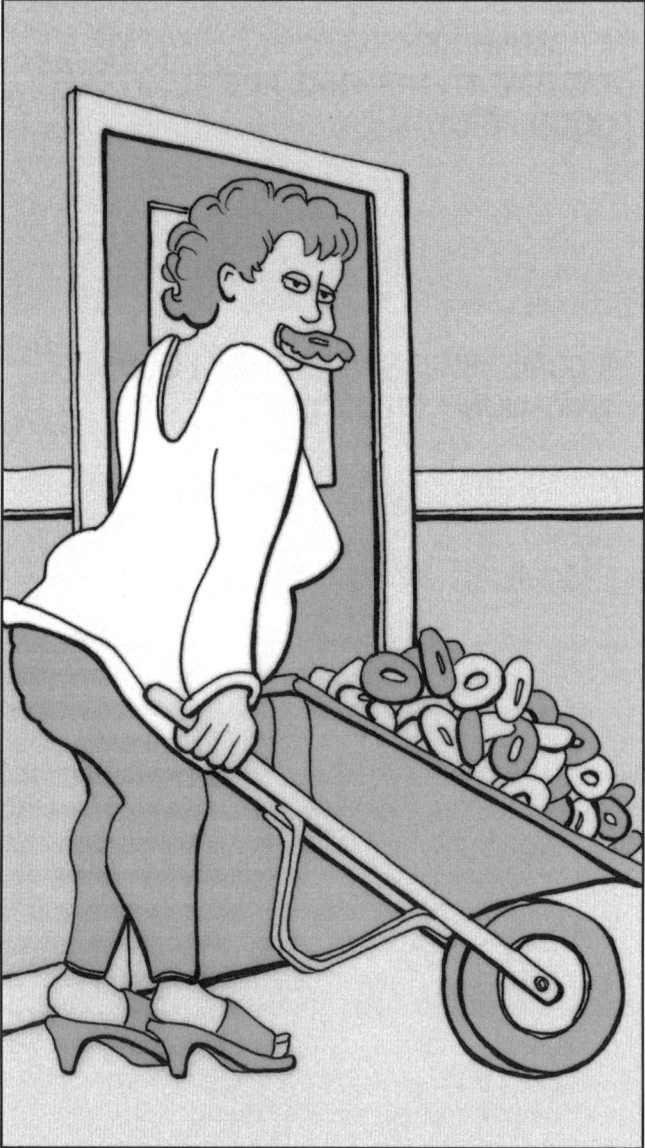

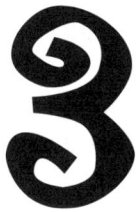

3 HOW TO CHEAT ON A DIET

Since there are so many people out there who are not familiar with Ben's Bogus Diet Breakthrough and the groundbreaking concepts of eating whatever they want and feeling guilty about it, many of the people you know, when you tell them you are dieting, will expect you to avoid unhealthy foods and get some exercise. Since this is a new concept, rather than confuse them, if you want to you can go ahead and act as though you are doing a more normal diet where you can't eat anything you like. Because those kinds of diets really stink, use some of the following techniques so you can eat the things you want. You may also want to share some of these methods with other friends of yours who are doing a more conventional diet and hating life.

20 TERRIFIC WAYS TO CHEAT ON YOUR DIET

Fill your belly button with frosting as you're getting dressed in the morning.

Feed your dog beef jerky, Spam, Vienna sausages or something else you like and snitch a bite or two when nobody's looking.

Start a food fight and when things get really out of control snag the good stuff out of the air.

At the restaurant, order a salad and low-cal glass of water, then excuse yourself to go to the bathroom. On the way catch the waitress and tell her it's your birthday.

Hide donuts inside your pillow at night.

Have false nails put on that are made out of pepperoni. Then all day long you can entertain your co-workers as you bite your fingernails and swallow them.

The bathroom is absolutely the best room in which to hide food. You can claim you're sick and go in there as often as you want, and if you make an occasional animal noise you can stay as long as you want... so long, in fact, that the food you hide in there and sneak can actually have enough time to cycle through. Then you can flush the evidence.

Fill your pen with whipped cream or grape jelly. No one thinks twice about pencil and pen chewers.

Carry your potato salad-filled shoes as though you were footloose and fancy free.

Keep as pets the types of animals you like to eat-a sort of "pet food storage." I'm sure that a halibut would look great in your fish tank and you know that rabbits, pheasants and turkeys are absolutely more trustworthy and make better pets than cats do anyway.

Replace your computer mouse with an éclair, PEZ or sausage McMuffin and pretend you're having computer problems.

Substitute frosting for your toothpaste when you brush.

Make up a story that needs acting out in which you use a pizza slice as a prop. For example, demonstrate how the dog bit someone - that someone can be represented by the pizza. Keep messing it up as you tell the story so you have to do it over and over again.

Distract your friends and slip a chocolate eclair underneath the lettuce in your salad at lunchtime.

Pick your nose and wipe the wrong finger on your pants. This leaves the edible protein based biodegradable material there for you to chew on later if you get hungry.

As you fill your blender with your diet protein shake, when no one's looking slip in a couple of donuts or some french fries.

Volunteer to take out the garbage, then pause for a while at the dumpster and root around in the junk to see if you can find anything good.

Send pork rinds or Twinkies to yourself in the mail. You can have them eaten before you get from the mailbox to the front door.

Wash a cinnamon roll down the drain, then later you can retrieve it by taking apart the P-trap.

While jogging, stick gummy worms to the shirt of the guy in front of you. If anyone gets caught cheating on a diet it will be him.

SINCE YOU'RE CHEATING ANYWAY

Here are some explanations you can use to explain why you continue to gain weight even though you're on a diet. These should mollify or at least entertain your harshest critics. Try 'em.

My doctor tells me I have a body type that absorbs calories from the sheets, blankets, and air around me while sleeping.

I'm not gaining weight; my friends are shrinking.

I'm being used for research. They're testing a new medication on me, which is intended to help anorexic people gain weight even if they don't eat anything.

I'm just ahead of my time. The sixteenth century style of chubby, fleshy women is making a comeback. I'm just one of the first to get in on it.

I have had these allergies that are really weird. Every time I sneeze hard, I blow up to the next pants size.

15

Those suppository laxatives I take turned out to be Heath bar miniatures. What a bummer. All this time I thought I was purging and instead I was eating Halloween candy.

Ever since I was hit by lightning my body has systematically begun converting carbohydrates into rare earth heavy metals.

Aliens are living in my abdomen. As soon as their babies hatch I'll look much skinnier.

Little fairy monkeys come in the night and slip French fries down my throat every time I inhale.

I have been constipated for the past three years. My body refuses to let even one calorie escape.

Last week my wife shaved my back and then oiled me down with some exotic massage oil she found in an Arabian flea market. About 5 minutes later my whole body, except for my ear lobes, swelled to three times its normal size. By the time the paramedics could shoot me full of steroids, I had developed an unnatural attraction to olives, which I have been eating by the handful ever since - especially the green ones stuffed with pimento. The good thing about the whole incident is that the exotic massage oil spilled onto a blanket which now floats around about three feet off the ground, which I use to get around until the swelling goes away.

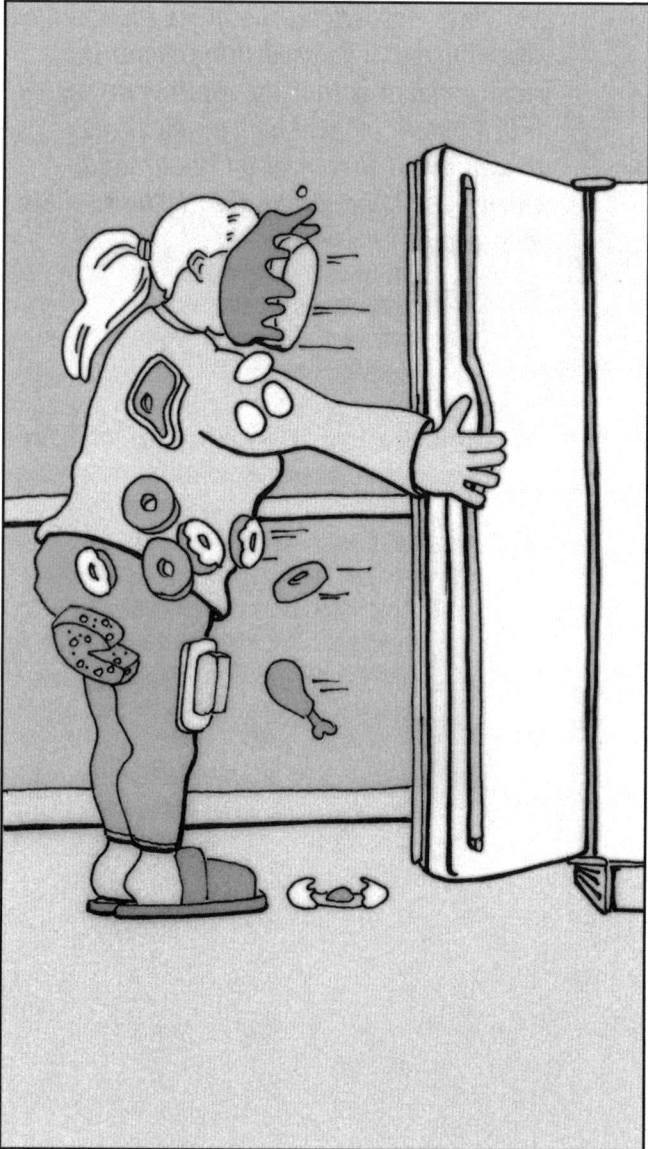

4 WHY WOMEN DON'T SEEM TO LOSE WEIGHT AS FAST AS MEN

I'm sure that many of you ladies have experienced something like the following: You look at your husband as he fills up the recliner munching bacon rinds, nacho chips, and Reese's Peanut Butter Cups. You need to lose a little weight yourself and get into shape, and so does your man. Since you know your slug of a husband won't do anything unless you lead him by the nose, you make a firm resolve, plan out a strategy, and bug your husband to join you in a fitness program.

On the appointed start date, the two of you wake up early in the morning and step onto the scales so you have a beginning point of reference. Then you eat a quick breakfast of celery and distilled water, while your husband has bacon and eggs, pancakes, and tops it off with Crunch Berries...and you're off for a jog.

The two of you run hard for what seems like a very long time. You come back into the house, tired, but contented, knowing you are working toward your goal. The curiosity is killing you, so you hurry back to the scales filled with anticipation. Your husband, on the other hand, suffering from a deplorable absence of curiosity, stops at the fridge for a cheese sandwich and pistachio nuts.

You step onto the scales and to your chagrin, you see that you actually gained two pounds while you were exercising. Wanting to make a point, you coax your husband into the bathroom to check his weight knowing that since he has been eating like a pig, at least you can take solace in the fact that he will have gained more weight than you.

He steps onto the scales. To your amazement, after only one workout he has achieved his target weight having lost 15 pounds in only thirty minutes of running. You conclude that this is not fair; you are cursed, and so you shuffle darkly back to the pantry and chug down a crate of cream puffs out of frustration.

Sadly, this scenario happens all too often. Maybe giving you an understanding of why will give you hope. (It might also give you the courage to finally kill the slug, but we will take our chances.)

WHY THIS IS SO

Women are made of sugar and spice and everything nice. Naturally, their bodies want to hang onto all that nice stuff. Guys, on the other hand, are made up of disgusting, smelly stuff, which their bodies want to spew out. So, all the while you ladies are exercising, your organs and tissues are grabbing and clinging to the good, wonderful things like the bagel and cream cheese you had for lunch the other day. At the same time your body is clinging to nice, sweet stuff, your husband's body is spewing filth. Run-spew, run-spew, and so forth. So, at the end of the day while your body has gathered up all these wonderful things and is clinging desperately to more of them than ever, your husband's body is relieved to be rid of a pile of disgusting, smelly stuff.

Don't feel bad, remember: God gave men stupidity to compensate. The question is, what can you do about it? Fortunately, you have Dr. Ben's Bogus Diet and Exercise Program. Forget about your man. Fight back. Start Dr. Ben's Bogus Program today without delay and you will feel better.

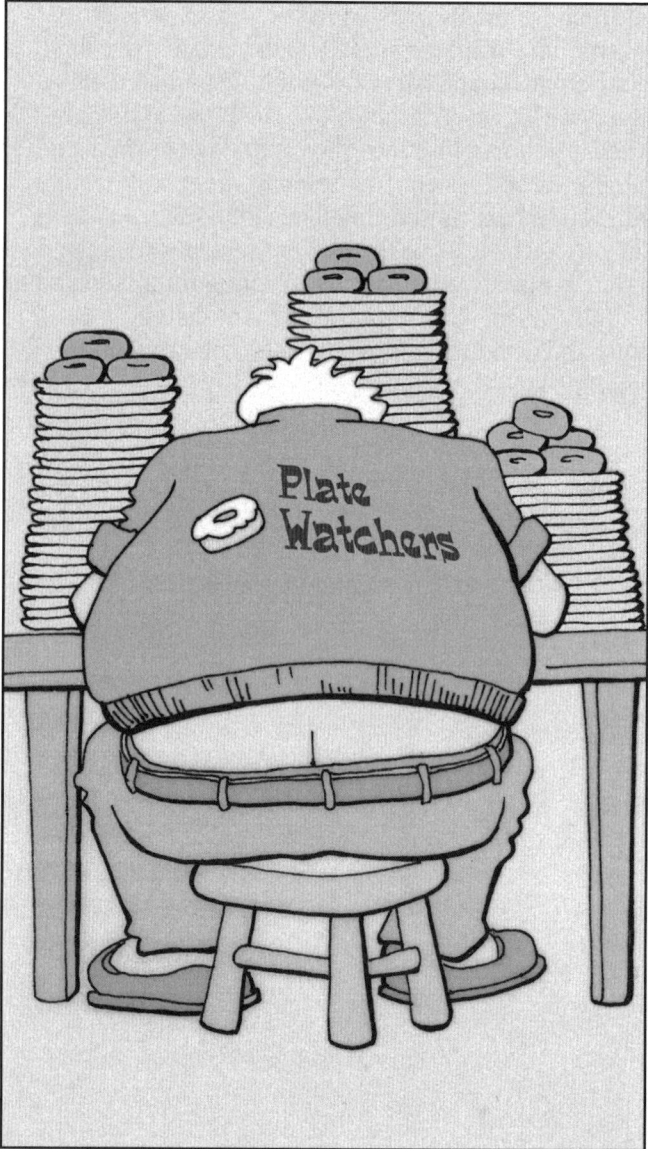

5 BAD DIETS

Sadly, there are unscrupulous people who will do anything for a buck. There are some real scoundrels and
creeps out there in the world who would rob you of
your health while fleecing you of your hard earned
cash. But, believe it or not, all of the creeps out there
aren't selling illegal drugs, and producing explicit
music videos and movies for your adolescent kids.
Some are also producing bogus diet programs.
Therefore, if you're going to run out and buy a bogus
diet book, we think you should definitely choose one
sold by only the finest people. If somebody has to get
rich promoting a bogus diet plan, wouldn't you rather
feel confident knowing that these are good, honest
people you're supporting? That's why with Dr. Ben's
Bogus Diet program, while, just like all the rest of

them, it's just a bunch of hooey, at least you can take comfort in knowing that we who are spending your money are pretty cool people, and, I might add, we are also really grateful for it.

Since even a bogus diet book ought to contain some useful information, to make us feel better about taking your money, we give you:

DIETS TO AVOID

**THE FOLLOWING ARE REALLY BAD DIETS.
DO NOT TRY THEM NO MATTER WHAT THEY
PROMISE OR HOW DESPERATE YOU BECOME.
ESPECIALLY YOU, CINDY!**

The Broken Glass and Gravel Diet

The Medical Waste Diet

The Excess Body Fluid & Mucous Diet

The Water & Amphetamine Diet

The Burrito Wrapper & Fast Food Container Diet

The Beef Tallow Diet

The Insect Repellent Diet

The Pre-Chewed Gum Diet

The Ex-Lax & Metamucil Diet

The Potato Chip & Beef Jerky Diet
(The author tried this in college)

The Tide & Mr. Clean Diet

The Construction Workers Dirty
Laundry Diet

The Pepsi & Mountain Dew Diet
(I tried this one in college, too.)

The Carp Counter's Diet

The Public Restroom Floor Diet

The Vietnamese Pot-Bellied Pig Diet

The Scab & Belly Button Lint Diet

The Ice Cream & Chocolate Diet

The Plate Watchers Diet

The All Bran and Beans Diet

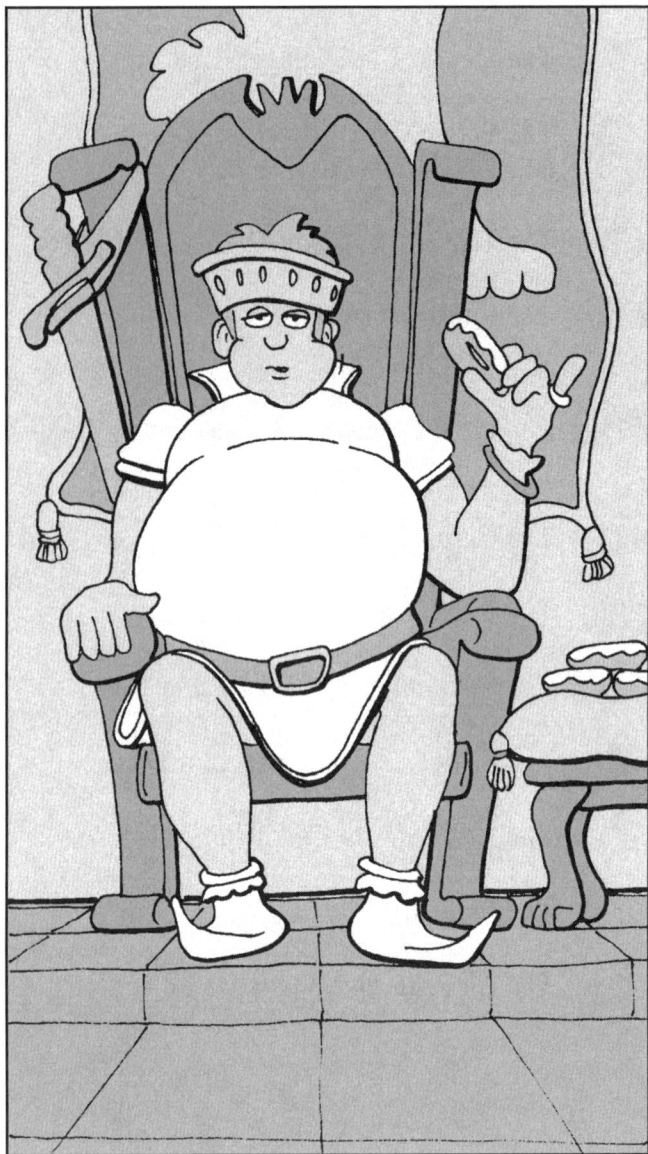

6 EXCUSES FOR NOT DIETING

After getting a look at those bad diets and knowing that there are many more dangerous diets out there that we failed to mention or even dream up, we offer you a list of pretty good excuses for not dieting, just to keep you safe.

13 Pretty Good Excuses For Not Dieting

You are storing up fat reserves for the great famine.

If you lose some of your mass your pickup truck will lose its good traction.

The healthy food terrorists out there who ruin everyone's day by warning about another favorite food that will kill us will win. You can't have that, can you?

It might be a very bad idea for the thin person who is inside you to get out.

Just think of all the good food that will just be wasted if YOU don't eat it.

What if you go to all that trouble and pain and then, popular fashion starts liking chubby people again?

What if you go to all the trouble of getting into great shape and become wonderfully healthy, but get hit by a garbage truck and die prematurely anyway?

What if you go to all that trouble and your friends don't like you any better?

What if you go to all that trouble and YOU don't like yourself any better?

Think of it. If everyone stops eating red meat, cows and pigs would very soon become extinct. Do you want that on your conscience?

If you really think about it, your best days are probably behind you anyway. Why shouldn't you blow up like a balloon if you want to? What else do you have to live for?

What's the logic of giving up everything that makes life worth living just so you can live longer?

Why bother? You know you will just blow it anyway.

What if you lose all the weight and then realize you <u>don't</u> have that pretty of a face?

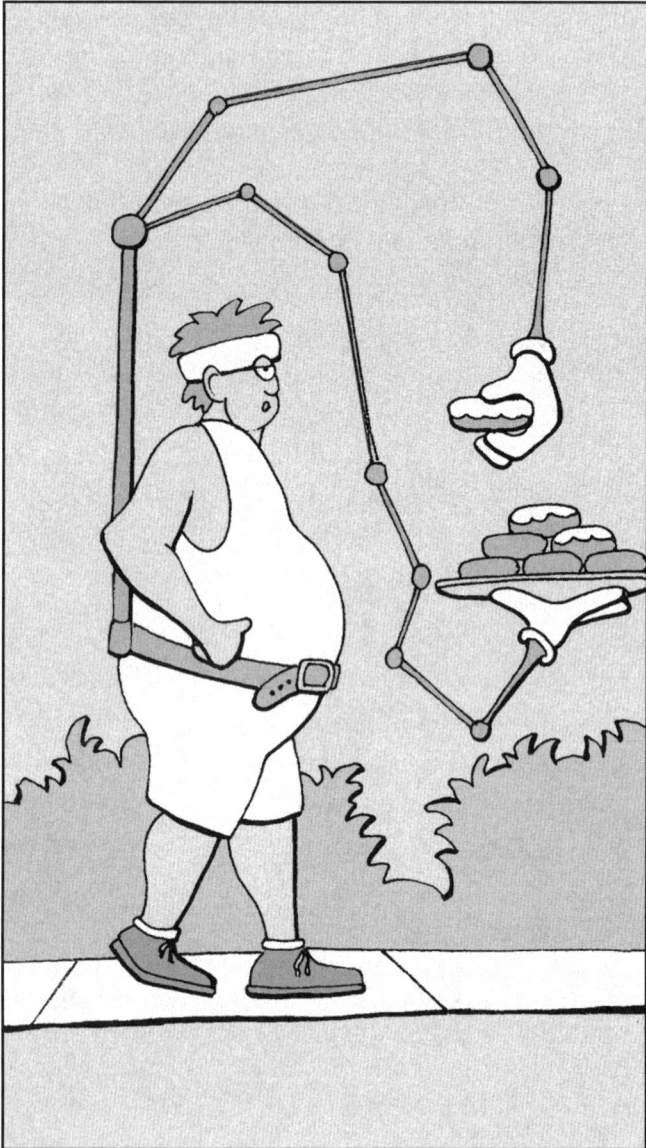

7 DR. BEN'S BOGUS EXERCISE PROGRAM

Exercise is a very controversial topic. Some of you get your exercise scratching under your armpit or coughing up a phlegm ball. This will not get it done. In this day we're all supposed to have buns of steel and a six-pack and look like we're eighteen when we're sixty. Besides, you know perfectly well that if you don't change behavior and quickly, you could find yourself dead from some degenerate disease... or even worse, still alive but looking like a bag of rocks in your spandex. This is why I recommend that you take your exercise seriously and this is why this chapter is in my book.

Now, when I say that I recommend that you take your exercise seriously, I don't necessarily mean that you need to do any actual exercise, at least not just yet. Let's not rush in to anything. What I mean by taking

your exercise seriously is just what I said, that you take
your exercise seriously. So, while you're being very,
very serious about exercise, I'm going to share a few of
my thoughts on the weather.

As many of you know, out here in The West the
weather is unpredictable. Those who have the greatest
understanding of this fact are those who try to predict
the weather, the local meteorologists (These are the
guys who should be out there predicting meteors or
something). They know from experience that they are
probably going to screw up their weather predicting
most of the time and so it looks to me as though they
have a strategy for hedging their bets professionally.
They cover all their bases. If you go to one weather
web site and look it will tell you one prediction, and if
you go look at another web site, that one will predict
something else. This system is terrific because with
every kind of weather known to man predicted on at
least one site, at least one meteorologist is bound to
be right at any given time. The added benefit of this
type of weather-predicting strategy is that it leaves
you, the weather-watching public person, to prepare
for virtually anything. In fact, it can also save you time
because you know that looking at the weather websites
is a waste of time because you know perfectly well that
the information is pretty much useless, and so you
save time by preparing for every possibility. Take your
sunscreen along plus your umbrella and a heavy coat
and gloves and swimming suit along with your warm
hat and boots.

This strategy is something that Dr. Ben recommends
when it comes to your health and exercise as well.

Because you never know what your body is going to do to you, when it comes to your exercise program, you better be prepared for anything.   For example, some people I know devote countless hours each week to working out. That's pretty much all they do. This class of people assumes that their body weather, so to speak, will always be good and healthy. Sadly, if all they ever do is prepare to be healthy and fit, they leave themselves unprepared and vulnerable for the possibility that their physiological weather will change to sedentary and sick-o, or even immobile and dead. What if, in the middle of their exercise regimen, the old obesity bug bites them hard and all of a sudden they become so heavy their joints can't take the pounding caused by running on the pavement. I know about this. It happened to me. What if some exercise buff is going along doing a regular workout and all of a sudden some disease like gout, plague, or sleeping sickness attacks and he can no longer do it?

That's why, just like the meteorologists, we recommend that you hedge your bets. If you want to work out a little, feel free, but don't put all your eggs in that cement mixer. Don't just beat around that particular fudge brownie. Also plan for the possibility that you might be unable or unwilling to exercise for a few decades. That's why Dr. Ben will never give you any specific exercise program. We're not going to risk telling you to go out wearing only your Speed-o and then have a snow storm move in, metaphorically speaking, and bury you under four feet of ill health. Take your exercise program very seriously, but at the same time, plan for attacks of inactivity, illness, and stupidity. That way you have all your bases covered.

DR BEN'S BOGUS EXERCISE PROGRAM IN TWO EASY STEPS

> **Step 1: Whenever you're really in the mood, do some exercise if you want to, or else don't.**

> **Step 2: Repeat step 1.**

Note: Most diet and exercise programs give you only one side of the debate: theirs. One of the unique things about Dr. Ben's Bogus Diet and Exercise program is that, in an effort to reduce liability, we try to anticipate some of our opponent's thoughts. So we present both sides. We want to be fair. So, in a spirit of cooperation and absolute fairness, we give you the other side of the exercise argument. Here go some pretty good excuses for not exercising that you really ought to consider before you start Dr. Ben's revolutionary breakthrough.

SOME GOOD EXCUSES FOR NOT EXERCISING THAT YOU OUGHT TO CONSIDER:

Some person you know (a good friend, relative, enemy, whatever) completely obsessed and knocked herself out getting in shape, exercising for hours a day and avoiding tasty foods for decades only to get hit by lightening just as she was approaching her ideal weight and fitness. You are determined this won't happen to you.

Fitness is just a fad. By observing Italian Renaissance art, anyone can see that throughout most of history, being chubby was a sign of beauty, wealth and prestige. Since every baby boomer has been a witness to the fact that virtually every fashion fad manages to cycle back around every few years, I'm going to wait until I can get in on that chubby one again. I can be patient.

If a person gets too much friction on his butt cheeks or where his legs rub together, there's a significant risk that a person's hemorrhoids could explode or burst into flames.

One needs to maintain all the mass one can in order to help his pickup truck get good traction.

Unfortunately, you are a person who is allergic to your own sweat.

With all the starving children in China, you can't bear the thought of wasting all those perfectly good calories just burning them all up for no good reason.

You know you would only blow it anyway.

DR. BEN'S BOGUS DIET BREAKTHROUGH

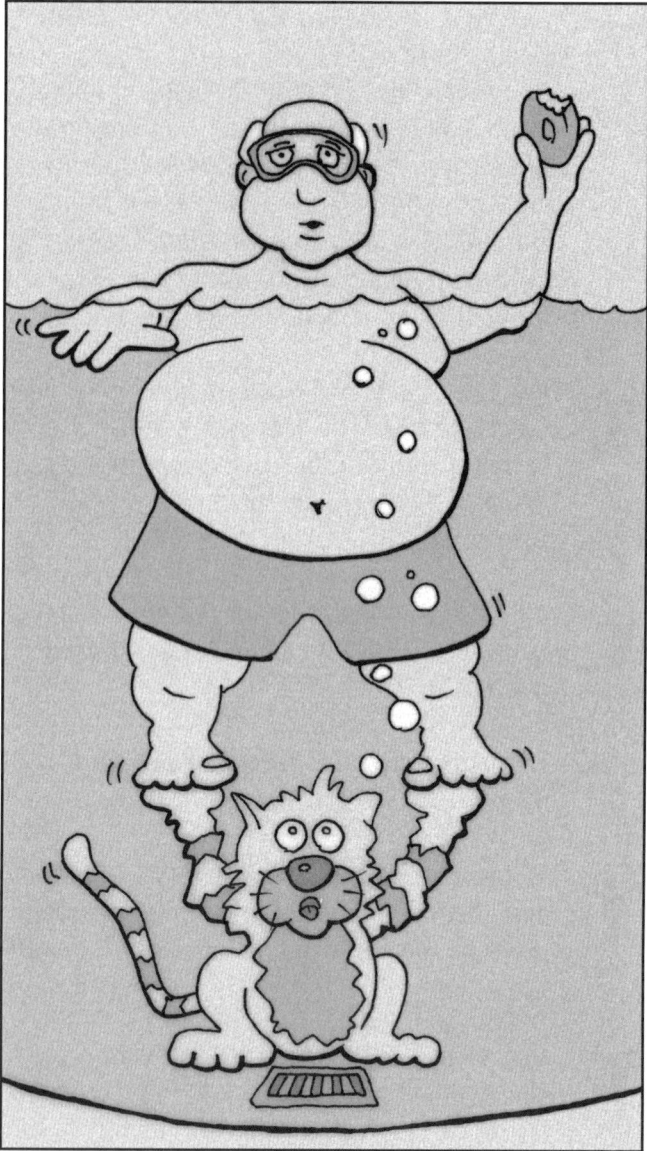

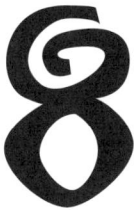

8 BALANCING YOUR DIET AND EXERCISE PROGRAM WITH THE HUMANE TREATMENT OF ANIMALS

According to some experts, the most important consideration on the minds of many diet and exercise fanatics is the humane treatment of animals. Apparently, judging from my mail, the most important thing on the minds of many skateboarders, serial killers, librarians, prison wardens, school teachers, dock workers, welfare recipients, mental patients and humor book readers is the humane treatment of animals. In fact, it looks as though that's pretty much all some people think about. I know this because occasionally, I have received letters from tender, caring, socially conscious individuals threatening to disembowel me, torture my grand children, and blow up my computer if I don't curb my enthusiasm for cat jokes.

Thus, it would be logical to conclude that, just like many humorists want to avoid offending free-speech-defending animal rights activists who would throw fire-bombs into their living rooms and chain themselves to cats and dogs, this would probably be a good time to observe that a very high percentage of my readers are committed to scrupulously avoiding any harm to animals during their diet and exercise experience; either that or else they want to provide the rest of us with a target group of people who take themselves way too seriously, and who are, therefore great to poke fun at. And since I don't know which group you, my incensed reader may fall into, and since I want to keep doing what I'm doing so I don't have to go out and get a real job, and since I also like my health and my grandchildren and our right to live, I feel that it is high time I did a bit of public service by providing some information about the protection of animal rights by health conscious individuals.

AS FAR AS I KNOW, NO ANIMALS WERE TORTURED OR ABUSED IN ANY WAY DURING THE PRODUCTION OF THIS BOOK.

As a public service, we hereby inform you that in order to avoid harm to animals, especially cats, you should refrain from buying any products, which include cat by-products or that were manufactured using methods which included the torture of cats. All such products should be clearly marked on the labels making identification pretty easy. Also, whenever you go jogging, walking, or cycling for your exercise and take along your cat, you should never chain heavy objects like land mines to her little feet or parade her in front of alligators or angry pit bulls. And of course you should note that because I am a super sensitive socially conscious kind of guy, since many humorists and diet book writers may not be, instead of writing caustic letters to me, you might need to really focus your attention on the other humorists. I suggest that the best way to get evil and insensitive comedians on board to your cause and to get them to stop making jokes about cats and dogs would be to figure out a way to acquire a sense of humor and to cool it with the righteous indignation, so you're not quite so much fun to tease. This would probably be a good idea for airport security personnel, traffic cops and Arab extremists, too.

Since I know that many of my readers are not too quick, some of them are a few marbles short of a full bag, the elevator doesn't go clear to the top floor, or, they're a hotel or two short of a mental monopoly, and will run right out and try everything I tell them not to do just because I told them not to do it, just as though they were one of my kids, so, in order to be sure we have none of that and to show that I am a stand up guy who wants to do my part to make cats and dogs feel more secure, here is a list of exercise and diet-related uses for a cat that would certainly be unethical. **STUPID PEOPLE, DO NOT TRY THESE!**

You should never swim laps using muffy as a flotation device.

It would be unethical to use muffy as a step-up during aerobic exercise.

You also should probably not use her as a sweat rag for your shoulders and armpits.

You probably shouldn't take Muffy jogging with you if the only reason you have her along is to be used as a distraction—to toss her behind you when a grizzly bear or pack of dogs comes after you.

If you happen to be going too fast down hill on your bike, don't toss muffy onto the road while she's tethered to the bike so she can dig her claws into the road as a drag in a futile attempt to help you slow down before you smash into that big rock or go flying off a cliff.

Don't spray-paint your animals to match your T-shirt.

And, whatever you do, don't ever use muffy to light the grill.

TIPS FOR APPEARING SKINNIER THAN YOU REALLY ARE

Rather than waste all those perfectly good calories by exercising them off, consider taking a completely different approach. Concentrate on ways of fooling people by making yourself look skinnier than you really are. Here are a few methods we came up with.

1. Wear tall, platform shoes, or better yet, stilts.

2. Wear big hair.

3. Get a job as a walrus or whale trainer.

4. Never be seen in person and whenever you talk on the phone try to sound skinny-inhale helium.

5. Do things to distract people so they won't notice your chubbiness: wear orange hair, have a sword poking through your tongue, or brain.*

*If you adopt this strategy you may run the risk of failing to distract the people from noticing your obesity and instead having them think you're whacked out. For example you may get comments like, "Hey, did you see that fat dude with the sword sticking through his head?" Sadly, there is risk in almost everything you do.
**OK, we admit this is a pretty short list. But, hey, this was a fairly hard topic. After straining our brain for longer than normal, these were still all the ways we could come up with at this time. Some topics are just like that. Life isn't fair.

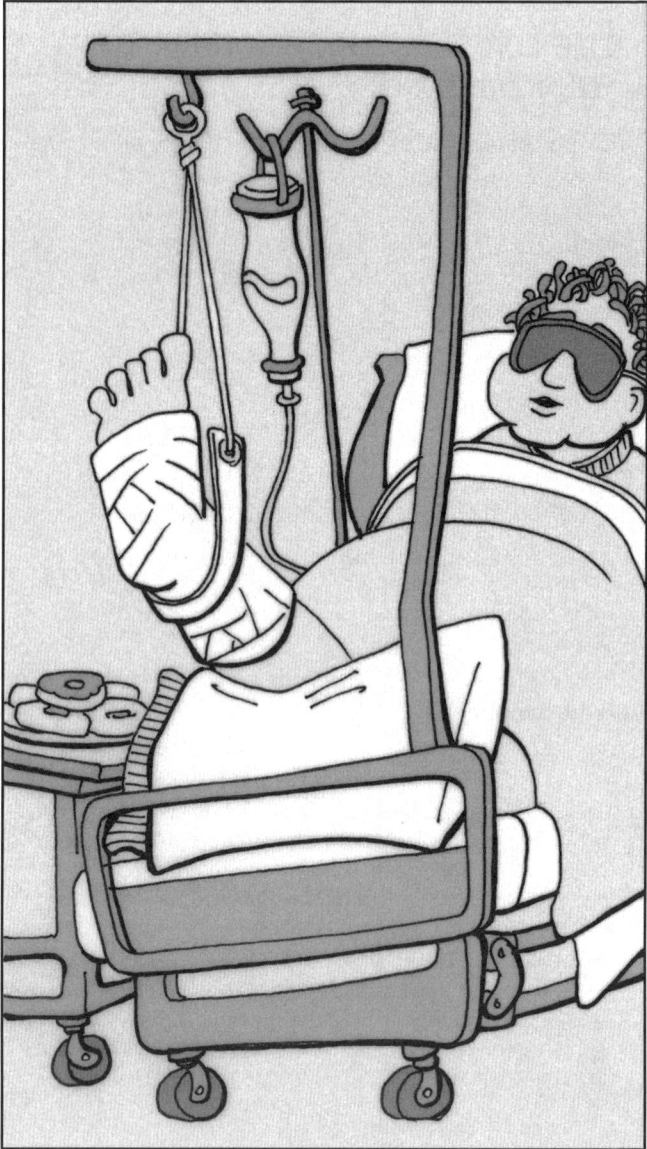

9

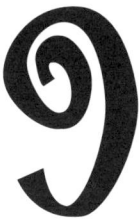

TACTICS FOR STAYING IN BED WHEN YOUR COMPANIONS ARE COMING TO GET YOU TO GO TO THE GYM, RUN OR WORK OUT

Poke gym socks up your nose so you sound stuffed up when they call and beg off because you have a cold.

Change our phone message to say you're vacationing on the French Riviera.

Tell them you were unable to sleep last night so you got up at 3:00 A.M. and did your workout already.

Get a big, mean dog. They'll mill around outside your fence for a while-maybe even call out to you, but if you ignore them long enough eventually they'll lose interest and leave.

As you're working out, talk politics or religion to them or better yet, try to get them into a multilevel marketing scheme. After that you'll never see them again.

As you're walking out the door, fake a sprained ankle. This may take a little practice, but it will be worth it. Then you can go back to bed.

Have a neighbor park an ambulance in front of your house with the lights flashing.

Wear a stereo headset with speakers pointing outward and play loud political attack ads, infomercials or kazoo music. This will act as a deterrent from ever being invited again. Next time they will tiptoe quietly past your house and hope you don't notice.

The night before, disguise or garble your voice as you call one of your friends on the phone posing as a terrorist and say, "We know your routine. You run every morning."

Rub your running clothes on a male goat's backside or cover them with doggie doo doo or fish heads and eat an onion and a couple of garlic cloves. If this doesn't get them to avoid exercising with you completely, at least it will allow you to trail behind and go at any pace you want to.

Eat a dozen scrambled eggs with cheese and drink a quart of hot cocoa, then open the door and throw up on them.

Here's one that will last for a month or longer: Have a fake cast put on your leg. This will also get you sympathy and considerable help in other areas of your life.

- PART TWO -

1 UNDERSTANDING EATING DISORDERS

OR, "ANOTHER INTRODUCTION TO THE PART OF DR. BEN'S BOGUS DIET AND EXERCISE PROGRAM FOR PEOPLE WHO BELIEVE THEY REALLY WANT A DIET OR EXERCISE PROGRAM"

Eating disorders are a big problem. We think you should definitely look out for eating disorders. Therefore, before you ever start a diet and exercise program such as this one, you need to be absolutely sure your head is screwed on straight. Specifically, experts insist that the key to avoiding eating disorders when you yo-yo diet, binge and purge, and otherwise abuse your body is to feel good about yourself. So, before you begin a systematic program of abusing yourself, make sure before you start that you have a healthy self-concept.

For most of us, the secret to feeling good about ourselves is to be healthy. Most of us are at our healthiest when we are fit, trim, and good looking. Experts[1] agree you should never begin a weight loss program when you hate yourself because your subconscious will just sabotage your efforts. You will catch yourself hiding from yourself and putting your finger down your throat after you eat, or going on a pure distilled water diet and then you will go home and eat your pets.[2] This would probably be a good place to note that most pet disappearances are not, as many would suggest, caused by alien abductions and auto-pet accidents. Most pet disappearances are caused by hungry dieters with a poor self-concept. The problem then is obvious. When you look really lousy and therefore feel rotten about yourself, this is not a good time to start a diet, which you will just blow in a short time and get fat and then feel even more rotten about yourself. So the times when you're fat and out of shape are clearly not the times to begin a diet and exercise program.

Before you start your diet, you must have a healthy attitude. The obvious way to do this is to look better than you do now. So before you start a diet or exercise program, consult your doctor and, of course, make sure that you have taken most of that excess weight off and you're in pretty good shape. Otherwise, the only rational diet and exercise program for you in your current condition is Dr. Ben's Bogus Diet and Exercise Program, which virtually anyone can do even if they are

in horrible shape and feel rotten about themselves.
And be real careful not to get any eating disorders.

[1] Doctor Phil, Oprah, and Sponge Bob
[2] Research into pet disappearances continues to be a hot topic
on late night radio talk shows along with crop circles and UFOs.

DR. BEN'S BOGUS DIET BREAKTHROUGH

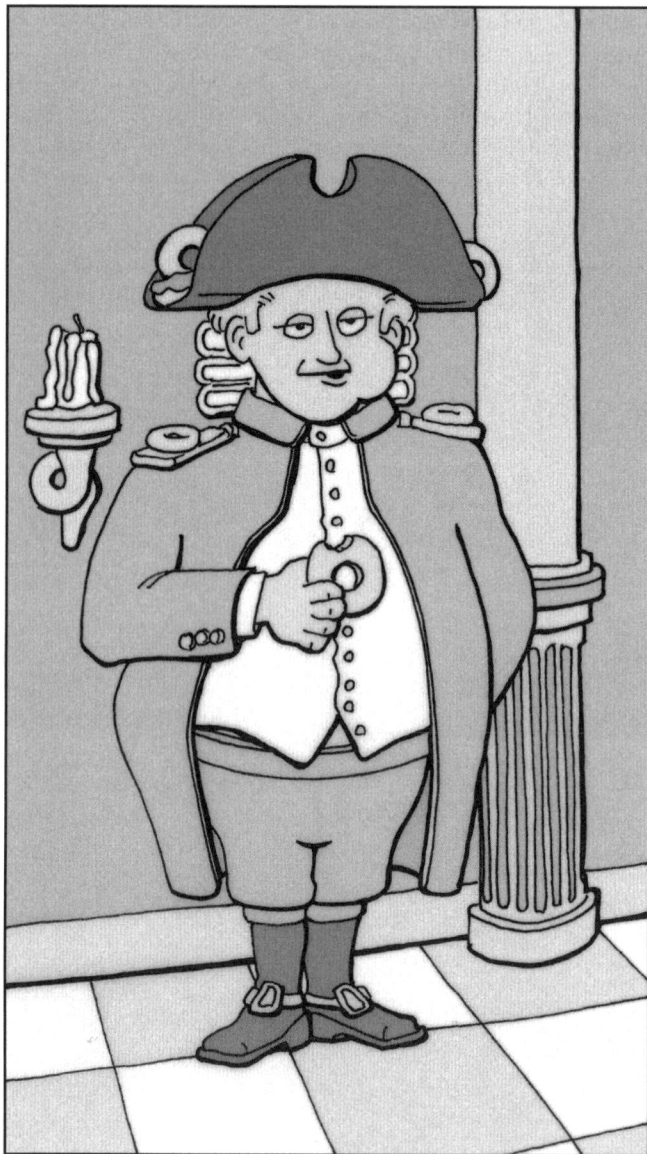

2 A HISTORY OF DIETING AND EXERCISE AS WE KNOW IT

A concern for diet and health has been with us since the dawn of history. Just like men and women of today, early man and woman wanted a healthy, fit appearance. In order to look fit and trim, many trendy cave dwellers explored innovative dietary options. Sadly, in the absence of consumer advocacy groups and ambulance chasing law firms, primitive man and woman were easy prey for unsavory promoters of trendy diet plans, which later turned out to be bad ideas and caused illness, premature death, age splotches, and stretch marks. With a limited hunter-gatherer style diet, most of these programs empha-sized foods rich in animal protein and low on carbs, which was actually probably pretty healthy if you don't take into account the high mortality rate from cave

bear attacks and mastodon hunting accidents. The
other main drawback was that this diet unfortunately
would have eventually caused liver and kidney problems, and enlarged prostate in consumers if life
expectancy had been over twenty-eight years. So, it
wasn't until much later, probably during the Bronze
Age, The Pax Romana, the Industrial Revolution, or
some other important sounding epoch that health-
conscious individuals discovered fruits and vegetables.
One can imagine some Roman making raviolis and
walking out into his garden while the noodles cooked
and shouting, "Hey, look! Zucchini! Leeks! Tomatoes!"

During the plagues of the middle ages, interest in diet
and nutrition waned due to a preoccupation with bur-
ial plots and scurvy, and so many people ate poorly
and didn't exercise. We see evidence of this trend all
over the place, since most of the women depicted in
Renaissance art are chubby and out of shape. Aside
from that, many of you noticed from your junior high
history books that they were also naked. Apparently,
many people who lived during the middle ages weren't
interested in clothes either, and since the times were
so hard, the health police were nowhere to be found.
Besides looking like a bunch of exhibitionists, you've
got to figure that people back then also had lots of
cholesterol and blood pressure problems along with
diabetes and terminal self-consciousness.

And so, time marched along, which marching made for
terrific cardiovascular health, at least in time, but
unfortunately, time was the only one getting any
healthier because men and women weren't exercising
hardly at all clear up until the French Revolution when,

thanks to Napoleon's concern that degenerative diseases such as obesity, high blood pressure, arrogance, and cowardice were showing up in French children earlier and earlier. Therefore, Napoleon's cousin, Covert Napoleon was assigned the task of improving the health of the children and aristocracy by coming up with a weight loss strategy which was just as effective as the guillotine, but which had fewer side effects. The best he could come up with was a land war in Asia, which turned into one of the first colossal diet debacles in recorded history culminating in a class action lawsuit which generated TV ads by concerned law firms that lasted nearly until the modern era.

THE MODERN ERA

Late in the nineteenth century, the exciting, new social, political, economic concept of Laissez Faire capitalism was gaining steam in the Western world. This resulted in an agricultural revolution providing what Teddy "F.D.R." Roosevelt described as a "chicken in every pot stirred by a big stick." This increase in available food, while increasing Americans' quality of life, alarmed many turn-of-the-century women because while surrounded for the first time by all that great food, their backsides grew so fast the only thing they could do was cover them up with petticoats and huge dresses. And so, suffragettes began to focus on diet and exercise with a real sense of urgency, with skimpy summer fashions just around the corner.

The first in a long series of fad diet and exercise books with titles such as Uncle Tom's Cal-burn and Gone With the Wind, were highly motivational and despite causing some real scary side effects, were financial mega-hits. And so, from that time, right up to the present moment, nearly every day we get at least one new diet and exercise breakthrough thrust upon us through the media. While many of us wonder on occasion what it is exactly that's "breaking through" we know that it's not the public's interest in diet and exercise books, because some pretty goofy and bogus programs have made millionaires out of thousands of unsuspecting shysters and hustlers. And so, this author is hoping that this trend continues for at least one more book.

MORE TIPS FOR APPEARING SKINNIER THAN YOU REALLY ARE

OK, I know that I said earlier that I had come to the end of my intelligence on this topic. However, I have since ran into a couple of experts on this topic down at Jack and Jill's Bowling Alley and picked up a few more tips while downing a double-chili, double-onion, double-dog with extra fries and a gutter-ball special.

1. Avoid wearing anything glossy. Matte textured clothes and accessories hide 'cottage cheese' bumps more effectively than items like disco-ball rayon shirts or vintage silk hosiery.

2. Wrap yourself in duct tape.*** This has the double effect of compressing flab and flaccid muscle into some semblance of a human figure while creating a vapor barrier that makes you sweat at 400% of your normal rate. You know you're done when you have sweat out so much salt and body oil that the duct tape doesn't stick anymore.

3. Try to only be seen in public at night and wearing matte black clothes. This works really well for movie stars who pack on the pounds between jobs.

***A note of caution here, this is not the best option if you happen to fall into the 65% of the general population who happens to be hairy and fat. It is a little known fact that the rapid extraction of body hair (in large quantities) may cause shock and require a hospital-based recovery.

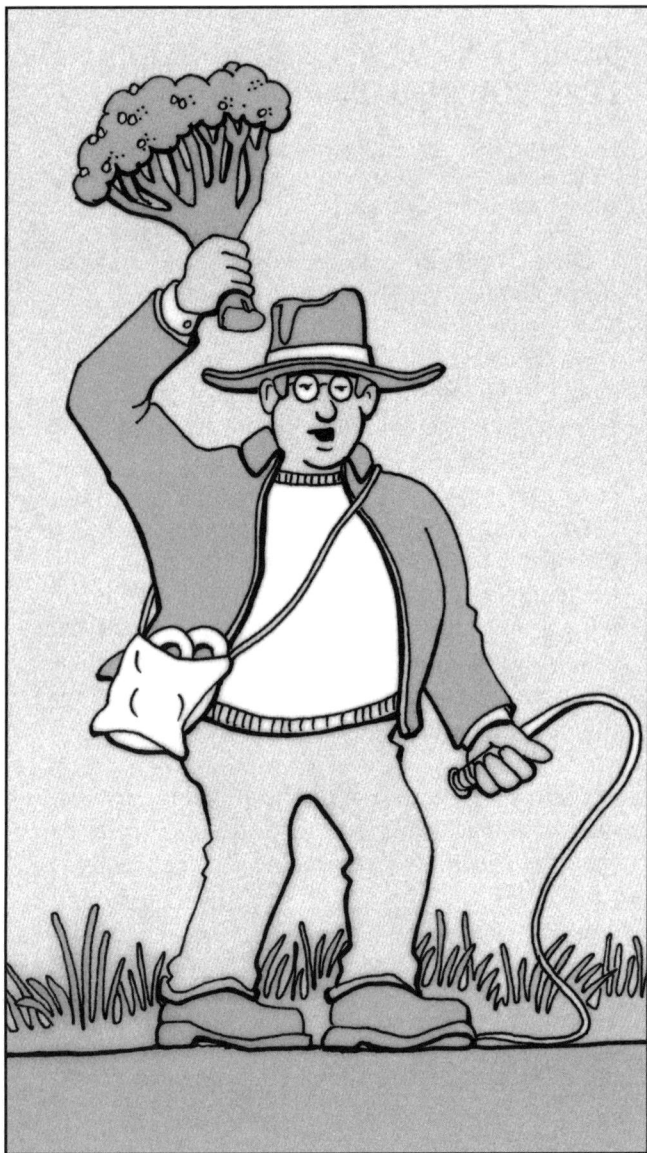

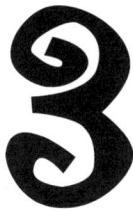

3 FOODS THAT WILL KILL YOU

Another ground breaking discovery this book dares to reveal is the truth that food will kill you, and I do mean ALL food. You know this from reading every magazine on the newsstand and from watching every news and news magazine show on TV. If you were to make a study of random diet and nutrition books, not only would you get so bored that you would probably want to take a job as seed counter just to get some action, you would also discover that in one book or another nearly every food known to mankind has been condemned as lethal to humans. As I tried to sort out what was healthy and what was not, at one time I came to the conclusion that good tasting food was bad and that nasty tasting food was good. And so I began to operate my life on the assumption. I ate nasty tasting foods regularly and on purpose, except every once in a while when I was really craving something good. After having eaten a whole lot of nasty tasting foods, I figured I deserved to eat something I liked. And so, I had peace of mind knowing I was eating healthy.

Unfortunately for people like me, science marched on. Since then, the food-health Nazis have succeeded in finding at least something deadly about even these lousy tasting foods. Therefore, we now know that not only will good tasting food kill you, but also that nasty tasting food can be just as deadly. Take for example the really really horribly awful tasting foods, the ones that rank a 10 on the nasty scale, the ones that are so disgusting that they make you gag just thinking about them, you know like, say, chubby grubs, caviar or eggplant. I'm sure that out there somewhere in the scientific world, some pinhead has done a study which shows that caviar will kill you, that if you were to inject extremely large amounts of caviar into the colons of hundreds of mice, for the first ten or fifteen years of this the mice would just get annoyed and wreak of fish, but as time goes on, say after twenty or thirty years, the mice would become snottier and snottier and eventually demand to wear little Abercrombie mouse clothes and drive a little mouse Lexus, and they would look down their whiskers at the rest of the animal kingdom. Such behavior would go on and on and even escalate until finally they were even too good for themselves. And so they would die of cancer. The same is also true of most other nasty tasting foods like Brussels sprouts and iguana livers when injected into rodents in large quantities. So much for the fiction that lousy tasting foods were healthy.

Still, we can't forget about good tasting foods. You
already knew that good tasting foods would kill you.
Root beer floats will cause you to become obese,
cheese balls will clog your arteries, Nerds will clean
out your sinuses leaving room for bacteria to multiply,
and everything out there causes rectal cancer. Some
foods will hasten a degenerative disease like arterial
sclerosis of the liver, Henderson's disease or prostrate
cancer. Stop dreaming of that food you're dreaming of
right now because, given half-a-chance it will attack
your heart like a thousand cholesterol ninjas.

The thoughts that all these foods that you like and that
you don't like are trying to kill you could cause depres-
sion, which will also kill you. Not eating any food will
cause anorexia, which we all know will kill you. What
is a garden-variety homosapien-sapien to do?
Fortunately you have this book to give you hope and
perspective. The next couple of pages have some
secrets to reveal that will finally give you clear understanding and offer some options that you can swallow
(No pun intended).

Since millions of dollars of research have proven that
nearly all foods will kill you, and since, in order to sell
our diet book we need some new information, however
inaccurate, to give the public an excuse to buy it so
they can have another fad, and we can rake in large
piles of dough, and since we really don't have any
good scientific research to fall back on, I am pretty
much left with my own uncannily accurate observations. I have observed two foods that, as of this date,
have never yet showed up on any real scientists radar
screen as being unhealthy. I don't know about you,

but I find it amazing that with all those millions of recipes and foods both ethnic and Republican that God made only two of them completely OK for human consumption. Amazing though it is, it could also be true. Maybe. And so we begin with the premise that this diet book is the only one ever written that fully divulges this great dietary secret. If you are human, the only two foods on the planet that will not kill you are: (drum roll please) those two foods are broccoli and tofu. I repeat: No one I know[1] has ever made the claim that broccoli and tofu will kill you. For heaven's sake, if these foods weren't safe, what other reason would they possibly have to even exist?

Disgusting, huh. However, with this knowledge you know that you have two choices. The first one is to make a complete life change to a strict diet of broccoli and tofu. The danger here is that for most of us who aren't little green worms, this diet would be more disgusting than actual death as far as we know[2]. And besides this, if my observations are correct, then a strict broccoli and tofu diet might cause a person to live to be very old. And since I've discovered that the older I get, the less tolerance I have for idiots, I figure that by the time I get to be a hundred and sixty I will probably get so annoyed by some particular idiot that I might actually kill him. This would be very bad because killing people, even idiots, is a major "no no" in most religions and so it would most likely send me straight to Hell. So the way I see it, the only way to protect the slim chance I have of going to Heaven is to pretty much avoid broccoli and tofu whenever I can. So I, personally, have decided against this first option. It's a religious thing.

The other option you have is to eat all the other foods you like in moderation and just figure that sooner or later as horrible as it may sound, you will die, if not from being killed by what you eat, from being run over by a garbage truck or something. And you should definitely stay away from experiments with mice and their colons.

[1] I should probably mention here that I don't get out much, so unfortunately, I don't know many people. Sorry.

[2] Sadly, there is still quite a bit of research to be done on death, as we know it.

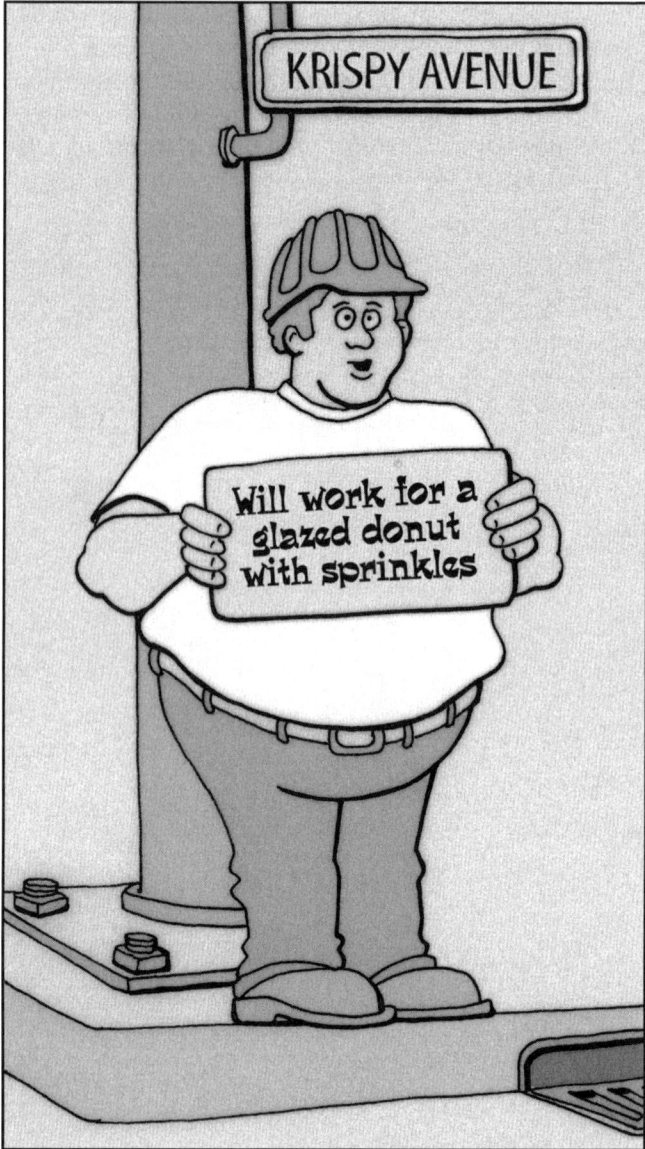

4 HOW TO MAKE MILLIONS IN YOUR SPARE TIME, GUARANTEED, WITH NO RISK AND DOING ONLY STUFF THAT IS FUN

In the year of Our Lord, 1977, I was about to graduate from college with a bachelor's degree in economics. I was pumped. I was all psyched up to go out into the world and make a million bucks in record time. I knew I was prepared. If you don't count the Psych class that was at 7:00 in the morning, the only classes I completely bombed were math and science; I knew lots of cool kids, and had been a pretty good football player, which, I figured, qualified me to do just about anything better than the old people and dweebes who were the most common variety of people running businesses out there in the real world at the time.

So, after a decade of having other people fail to recognize my potential and neglecting to give me the tons of money I figured I was worth, I was beginning to wonder if I missed the class in college that explained the part about getting people to pay me what I was worth. Maybe I was even beginning to lose a little confidence. So, at about this time, in an effort to build my self-esteem, I became a writer. This allowed me to go out and experience some serious rejection. So, if we skip over most of the mundane, common, and embarrassing stuff that happened in my life, this gets us up to the time a few years ago when I went back to school to see if I could find the class about getting rich that I had missed on my earlier try. At the time I was making really big bucks teaching high school English and writing part time for a small town newspaper. Naturally, since nearly 0.5% of new businesses make it past the first 2-years without going under, I knew the time was right to start my own publishing business.

STARTING MY OWN PUBLISHING BUSINESS

So, for the next 10 years I survived owning my own business and in the process defying all the odds, thanks in part to an uncanny ability to live for a month on the amount of money the average American family wastes on vegemite, and to block out of my mind gathering clouds of economic doom, which got me to the point where our company needed a mission statement. Well, at least, that's what the experts all told us at the time. So, we went to work on a corporate mission statement. The problem in our company was that there were two of us. And one was my wife, Robyn, who has an overdeveloped sense of basic character and integrity, so she tended to veto every functional mission statement I came up with. After eliminating the inaccurate or potentially misleading ones, we were left with these, which unfortunately very accurately described our true mission as we saw it at the time.

OUR MISSION:

1. To persuade our creditors to back off. If this wasn't possible, then to distract them long enough for us to get them partial payment.

2. To build up enough "good will" to become the target of frivolous lawsuits.

3. To try to get someone else to do the really unpleasant things necessary for our business to succeed.

4. To find ways to make real fun activities produce some revenue.

Anyway, we decided that maybe corporate mission statements weren't the answer for our little company, so we had to come up with another strategy. We decided to try writing a book on how to get rich. Figuring that we have such vast experience, since we have eliminated more unsuccessful possibilities than most people, we could consider ourselves experts and have our agent get us on talk shows. Sadly, all we could come up with on the topic of getting rich was this chapter, and not wanting all that work to go to waste, and figuring that the whole reason why we wrote this book on diets and exercise was to get rich so quickly that we would be long gone before people got sick and sued us over the bogus diet, we decided to include this chapter in our diet book. We have some wonderful, faithful readers who we figure deserve to get rich as much as we do, so we decided to let all of you in on the deal too. To that end, we offer you:

FOUR EASY STEPS TO GETTING RICH SELLING DR. BEN'S BOGUS DIET AND EXERCISE BREAKTHROUGH

Step #1 Order 10,000 copies of **"Dr. Ben's Bogus Diet and Exercise Breakthrough."**

Step #2 Make a list of all the people you know who have poor judgment or who have been known to make occasional ill-advised purchases.

Step #3 Contact each of those people and promise whatever it takes to get them to buy at least one of the books.

Step #4 Put the unsold portion of the books in the garage while you seek further inspiration about what to do with them and invest your profits in mango futures.

GOOD REASONS TO START A DIET

1. You feel some twisted need to punish yourself.

2. You are sick and tired of eating luscious foods and rich desserts.

3. You have never tried a diet and before you die, you want to have that experience.

4. You are looking forward to the time when you finally blow your diet again and you get to go shopping because you have gone up one more pants size.

5. Lowering your blood sugar while you greatly increase your hunger pangs will make you a happier person.

6. Somebody has to be a statistic. In a few years when this particular diet craze is held up for ridicule because it has been proven to kill you, one of the statistics might as well be you.

7. You want to do your part to improve living conditions in the world by supporting the poor people in the diet industry.

8. You want to do your part to save the earth by reducing consumption of plants, animals, and minerals.

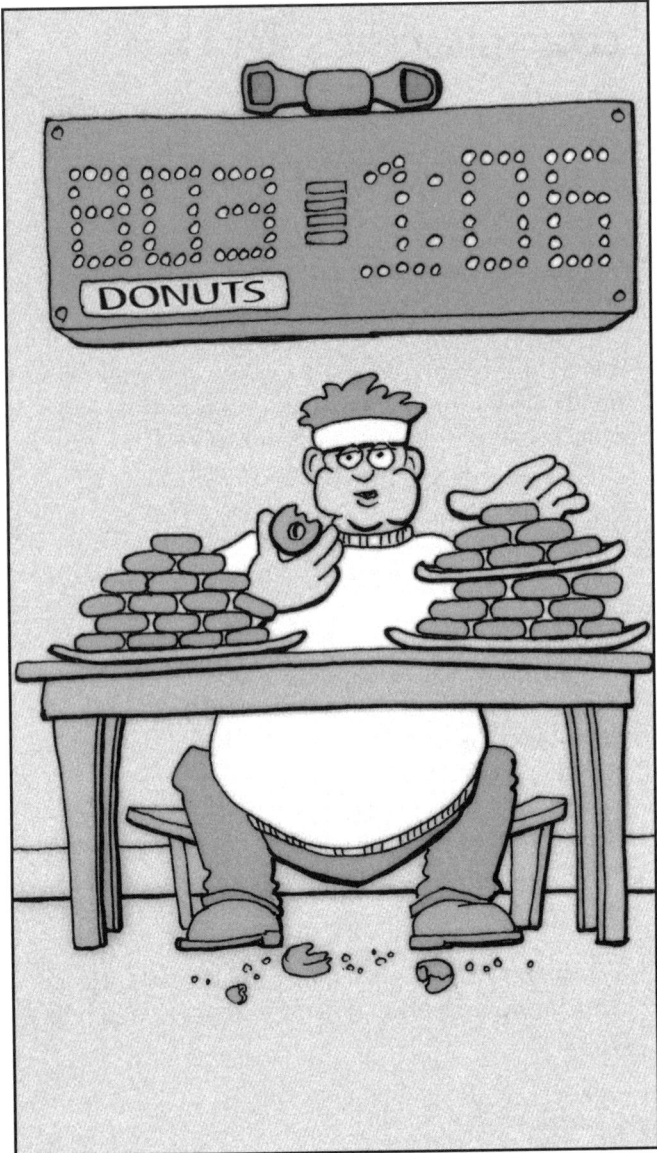

5 THE ROLE OF COMPETITION IN YOUR BOGUS DIET AND EXERCISE PROGRAM

When I was a teenager, my friends and I did what most teens do—tried to see how stupid we could be and still survive. One of our favorite activities was "beat the train to the crossing game". While there are probably many child and adult advocacy groups out there who would frown upon our old 'beat the train to the crossing' game, still, I believe there are times when competition like this can be a healthy thing.

Take dieting and weight loss for example. Many of us benefit from a little friendly competition: Competing to find out who can lose the most weight in a two month period without methamphetamines or lopping off a body part, can often improve results or increase frustration. Take running for example. Sometimes a person can get in shape faster by competing with another runner to see who can be the first to become permanently disabled from terminal shin splints, thus getting to the end of an exercise program faster than otherwise possible.

We know that some of our readers are not too creative and since the beating the train to the crossing game is a little dangerous, we would like to suggest a few less dangerous competitions: You might try "beat the pedestrian to the crossing," which can have much less painful consequences if you lose or, better yet, "Beat the cat to the crossing," which has only happy consequences as far as we know.

Another good opportunity for friendly competition is in the area of eating right. As you know, grains are good for you. You probably want to eat lots of grains. Wheat is a grain; flour is made from wheat, and Krispy Kreme donuts are made partly from flour. Why not have a competition to see who can eat the most Krispy Kreme donuts or, if there's no one worthy of your competition just see how many you can eat all by yourself. In fact, there's probably a Guinness Book of Records record for donut eating if you're really motivated.

As a kid, watermelon was also very important in my life. My cousin, Ray, and I used to have competitions to see how much watermelon we could eat. Sometimes we would eat so much watermelon we would throw up, and since calories have a hard time attaching themselves to our thighs when they are being chased through the air at 70 miles per hour by peas, corn particles and gastric juices, it seems to me that watermelon competition could be good, too.

Now, I know that there is a growing movement in this country away from competition. Many people in our school systems are working to find activities that discourage competition in order to make those students who are too lazy or incompetent to compete feel better about themselves. Some advocates go so far as to suggest that we eliminate grades altogether.

Fortunately for you, Dr. Ben's Bogus Diet was designed for either group. Whether you are in favor of competition or if you are a total loser, you can still be successful at this diet.

Even if you're totally not into competition, anyone can readily tell just by looking at you that you need motivation. Looking better, feeling better, and living longer are ideas that obviously are not working for you. You need something better to motivate you. Here are a few ideas of thoughts, which might do the trick for special cases like yours.

THOUGHTS TO MOTIVATE NON-COMPETITORS

Thought #1: By dieting you'll be doing your part to alleviate hunger in the world (except yours, of course). You're saving food so there will be more left for starving people in Afghanistan or China, Ethiopia, or for anorexic magazine models.

Thought #2: When you begin exercising in earnest, you will find that you are exhaling additional carbon dioxide, which plants love, thereby supporting ecology and increasing greenhouse gas emissions.

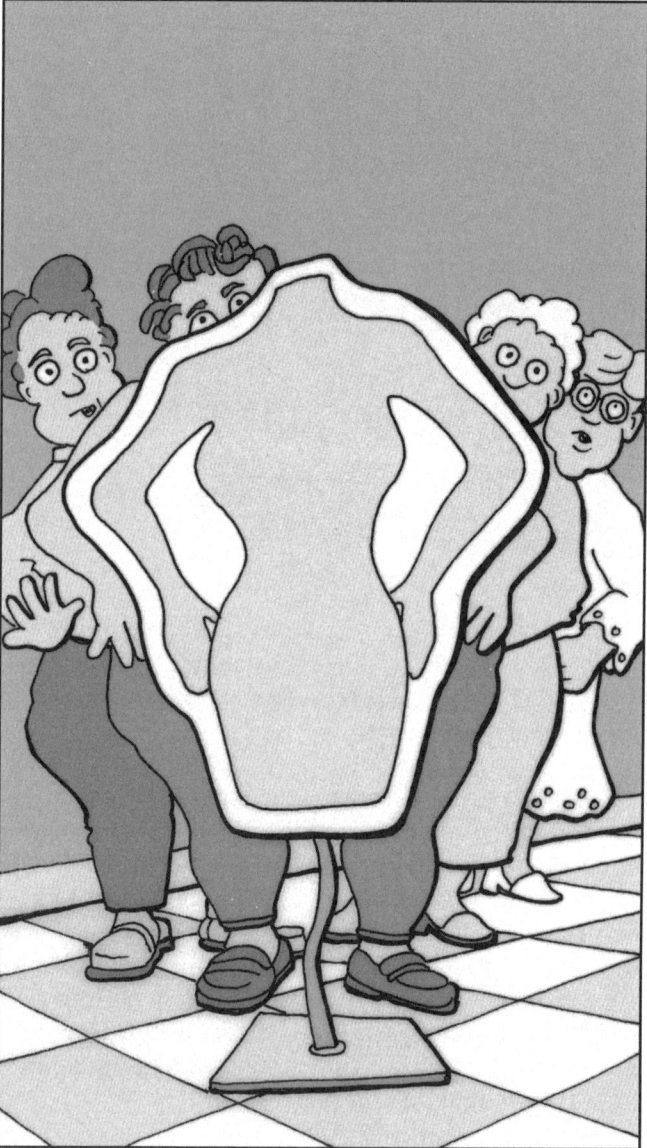

DR. BEN'S BOGUS DIET BREAKTHROUGH

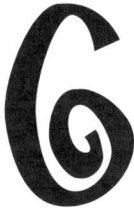

6 BIG FAT IMPORTANT TIPS

HOW TO BRING OUT THE SKINNY PERSON INSIDE YOU

When it comes to exercise programs and diets, throughout my lifetime I have jumped into them with a level of enthusiasm normally only seen at summer walrus colonies and in lines of school children waiting for measles shots. Thus, I have fallen a little behind some of my more committed colleagues-roughly 50 years behind. This has led me to ponder why it is that some people are skinny and some are not. What causes one person to become so focused that she exercises 3 or 4 times a day, avoids eating food for sometimes months at a time, often putting her finger down her throat when food accidentally finds its way in there until eventually she is mistaken for a viper and is eaten by mongoose; while at the same time another person gets most of his exercise scratching under his arm pit, tanks up on pork rinds, Big Macs, and Krispy Kreme Donuts despite warnings from his doctor that he may be eaten by hikers who mistake him for a giant fungus. So we see, there is quite a contrast between persons when it comes to their commitment. Why is this so, you ask? Attitude is the answer. Whichever side you happen to fall on, you can blame it all on your attitude.

HOW TO CHANGE AN ATTITUDE

The key to having the body you have always dreamed of, or the key to liking your frumpy body is your attitude. So, if you are one who doesn't like your current attitude, let us here at the institute for diuretic research help you change your attitude.

Let's say you are one of those who is way too into diet and fitness and your only friends are your athletic trainer and therapist. You carry your lunch to work and all you have in your pail are two Ex-Lax squares, a beaker of water and a Fitness magazine. You're beginning to fear being mistaken for dental floss, and you feel it's time for a change. You know the key to changing is finding a way to feel all right about having a frumpy body, to being perfectly OK knowing that your cholesterol, blood pressure, and weight are high and your stamina is low, so you can try something different for a while. Here's what you do:

HOW TO LOSE 2 POUNDS IN 5 YEARS

As we have already pointed out, the secret to good weight loss is attitude, or perspective, if you will. The average person gains a little weight as he or she grows older. This is perfectly natural. For example, between the ages of 30 and 40, the average woman in America gains 9 pounds. So, the way I figure it, if you were one who only gained 4 pounds, and, assuming you do math the way the government budget office does, you would have a net loss of 5 pounds! All this success occurs just when you do what you would normally do anyway. We call this particular diet, "The Government Math Corollary to Dr. Ben's Bogus Diet" and nearly anyone can succeed at it.

I know what some of you are thinking already. You are saying to yourselves, "Yeah, that's all well and good if you only have a little bit of weight to lose, but I have gained 250 unwanted pounds. 5 pounds is just a drop in the bucket. What can your diet do about that?" I would say to that, never underestimate the creative power of hungry politicians wanting desperately to get elected. Remember a few years ago you were out of work, the economy was in the tank, and your elected officials were crowing about having created 3,000,000 new jobs. When you heard that, you thought to yourself, "Do these guys live on the same planet I do? Everybody I know has their kids up for sale to pay the mortgage. Where did they create these jobs, for aliens?" And your thinking would be right on the money, because they actually were transferring millions of jobs to aliens, offering benefits to aliens and in general making life much better for aliens. Now that you know this, you can use this same government technique to lose your excess weight, even if you need to lose a lot of weight.

For example, let's say you are seven hundred and fifty pounds overweight and someone else has to tie your shoes for you. You would like to get that weight off, but doing what those other legitimate diets want you to is wretched and miserable, you choke down lousy food, or starve while grinding out brutal exercise regimens. You want no part of any of that. The way for you to get that unwanted weight off is the same way your elected officials do: take credit for someone else's weight loss on paper. Just find someone else who has lost the 30, 40, or 50 pounds, even if they happen to be an alien or if they lost it because they contracted colon cancer, and then, using the same principle as the government, announce to the world that the weight has been lost. Then, you can be firm in the knowledge that you are sort of telling the truth after a fashion, because the weight was indeed lost and is not likely to be found by anyone who will incriminate you.

OVEREATING

Overeating is another real problem. Today in America, good food surrounds us. Like 500 hogs in an Egyptian brick pit after the monsoons, we are literally wallowing in food. And so it should come as no surprise that like an adolescent gerbil in a grain silo, many of us consume twice our weight in food each day. Many of us eat like a polar bear just out of hibernation.

But we should bear in mind this was not always the

case. Historically, many people lacked enough food to even survive. Why, I remember my grandpa telling stories of going to bed hungry and having to outwrestle the dog for a rancid coyote pelvis for his supper. Today, however, thanks to the amazing engine of American free enterprise, virtually no one in this country lacks the basic essentials of life: food, clothing, a house with two TVs, a VCR, a cell phone, two cars, a computer with the internet, and an ex-wife or husband, so we tend to overindulge somewhat in the eating department.

Again, the secret to controlling our overeating urges is attitude. Since we are constantly surrounded by yummy things like German chocolate cake, Italian sausage, Reese's Peanut Butter Cups, hamburgers with cheese, potatoes and gravy, bacon, eggs, hashed browns, and pancakes, moose tracks ice cream with hot fudge topping and whipped cream, we might as well just bag this diet stuff and go grab something to eat.

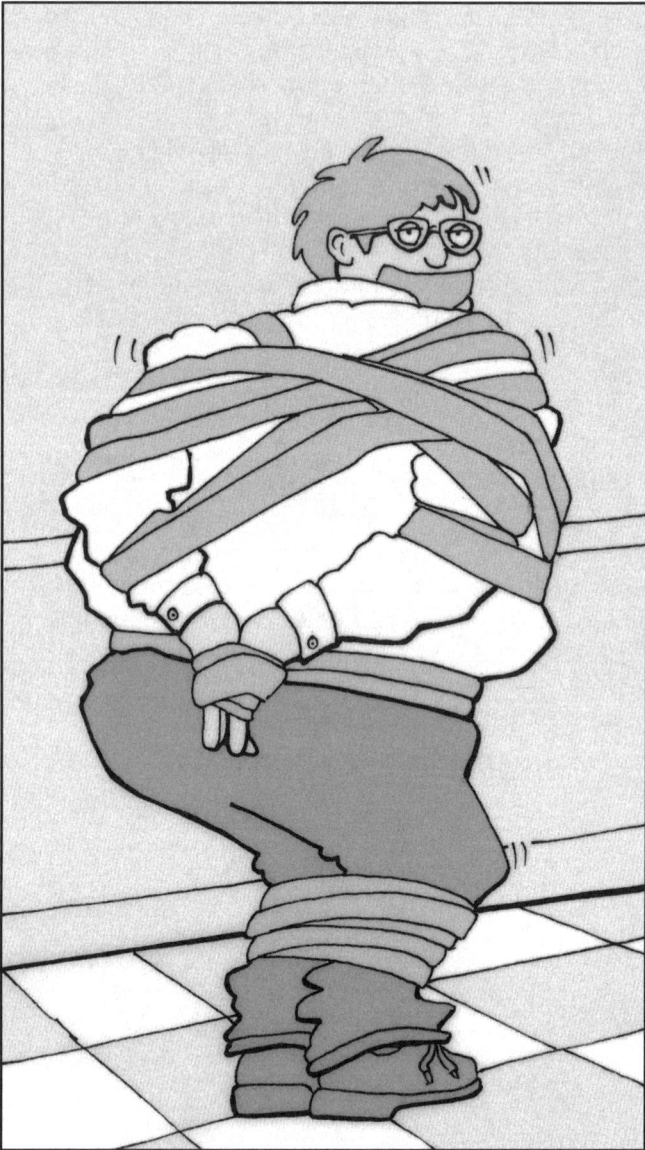

7 HOW TO FORCE SOMEONE YOU LOVE TO DIET OR EXERCISE

At one time or another nearly all of us has taken a look at someone we dearly love and thought to ourselves, "Gag! You look disgusting!" Whenever you find these thoughts popping into your head, especially about a spouse, it's probably time to manipulate your loved one into some kind of a trendy diet and exercise program.

Naturally, the easiest way to do this is to somehow convince him or her read Dr. Ben's Bogus Diet and Exercise Breakthrough. Even the least motivated of your loved ones should get excited about following OUR program. The problem with this is that after a few months of rigorous devotion to the diet, he or she will still look pretty much just as revolting as before and if you truly do want to get them to do something which will actually make a difference you may have to go a different direction. First, it's important to us that you know that we're OK with that. We know that our program, while it certainly is revolutionary and ground breaking, doesn't work for everyone. For you, it may be time to pull out all the stops and come up with some ways to motivate your significant other to do something about that disgusting body.

I'm amazed at how many of life's problems can be solved by hearkening back to simpler times. Remember back to your high school days when the Driver's Ed instructor would fire up the old sixteen millimeter projector and show a few hours of death and carnage, blood and guts in order to motivate you and your friends to be safe and responsible drivers. By the time this was over you were all the most cautious and responsible drivers on the road—right, and about that time, chickens could yodel and Boars could have babies. Of course that tactic didn't work. You all went out and did what you always did: let the car pretty much drive itself while you and your distracted friends fought over who got to change the radio station. If anything, this shock tactic had the opposite of the teachers' desired effect.

"What does all this mean?" You ask. Actually, we're not sure either. If we had any useful information, we would be curing colon cancer or winning a Pulitzer Prize in molecular physics not writing a bogus diet book, but the one thing we do know is that this tactic didn't work and it may have actually influenced rebellious teens to even be more irresponsible. We should also probably consider that it is entirely possible that this result was actually planned, that after spending a semester with us, our driver's Ed instructor and other teachers may have hated us so bad that they actually hoped these films would motivate us to go wreck our cars and kill each other, thereby leaving more room on the road for him and the other teachers. You really have to consider that this might actually be the case. But the thing we can learn from hearkening back to this experience is that it is indeed possible to influence others' behavior.

The problem is that normally when we do influence others' behavior we're not aware that we're doing it; however, the best way to try to make a difference, especially with other adults, is through the use of child psychology. You do this by hammering on them to do the opposite of what you really want them to do. Since we really are not qualified to teach you detailed psychological methods and techniques, after all, this is a bogus diet and exercise breakthrough, it's probably better that we stay with something we're more qualified to do. The one thing we are qualified to do is tell jokes, which, unless they are ethnic slurs have very little liability, so here goes:

Q: What did one dehydrated Frenchman say to the other dehydrated Frenchman?

A: What do we do now, Pierre? (pee air)

Anyway, we hope you liked it, but back to the problem at hand, if you really are serous about getting your slug of a spouse to lose some weight and get in shape, we know people who have tried shame, ridicule, positive reinforcement, social pressure, disease, fear, threats of physical harm and terrorism. None of these seemed to work unless the spouse had a naturally high metabolism, firm muscles, and long legs. So, the way I figure it, if you chose to marry someone with soft muscles, short legs and a slow metabolism, you pretty much have no one to blame but yourself. So I say, bag it and join 'em in front of the TV.

"Without Food"

(Sung to the tune of "Without You" originally by Badfinger or Harry Nillson, but most recently sung by Mariah Carey, or some lady like that with a big voice.)

NO, I CAN'T FORGET LINGUINI
OR YOUR CHEESE AND FETTUCCINI
BUT I GUESS THAT'S WHY MY SIZES GROW AND GROW
I BUY CHEESE FRIES UNTIL THEY'RE COMING OUT MY NOSE
AND IT SHOWS

NO I CAN'T RESIST THE JELL-O
SO I'LL TRY AGAIN TOMORROW
I'LL BAKE SOME COOKIES
THEN I'LL EAT THE DOUGH

NO FAIR THAT SOME CAN EAT THE WHOLE KABOODLE-0
AND STILL NOT SHOW

I CAN'T LIVE
IF LIVING IS WITHOUT FOOD
I CAN'T LIVE
I CAN'T STARVE ANY MORE

I CAN'T LIVE
IF LIVING IS WITHOUT FOOD
I CAN'T LIVE
I CAN'T STARVE ANY MORE

NO I CAN'T FORGET TOMORROW
'CAUSE TEN DOLLARS I WILL BORROW
I'LL BUY SOME TWINKIES
AND SNARFF SOME OREOS

I'LL EAT THE BAGELS 'TILL THEY'RE COMING OUT MY NOSE...THEN SOME ROLLS

I CAN'T LIVE ETC...

TESTIMONIALS

Of all the diet books I've read in the past few hours, I am convinced that this one has the best chance of becoming a fad and making the author a big pile of money.

E. McMahan

Over the years my cellulite and I have become such close friends that I truly don't want to get rid of it. That seems so harsh. This plan lets me keep my good friends.

M.R. Rogers

This is the only diet and exercise book I've ever read that didn't defy the laws of physics.

Al Einstein

I've gained 15 pounds this month and after reading this revolutionary book, I don't even care.

A. E. Newman

For a bogus diet book author, Dr. Ben truly has an intriguing philosophy.

Plato

I was really glad to hear that no cats were harmed in the production of this book.

Peta Pan

If I had found this book before I tried all those other really bad diets, I might still be alive today.

Socrates

At our house we have been using the book to hold the lid down on the gerbils' cage so they can't get out.

Bob

Before I found Dr. Ben's Bogus Diet Breakthrough, I was broke. I read the chapter that explained how to use the book to make money and I followed the steps as outlined. While I didn't make any money, and while I did annoy a few of my friends, I did succeed in having a big pile of books in my garage, and you can too!

Ben Vagrant

Having bought other diet books which promised good ways to cheat on a diet, I have to say that compared to all the other bogus diet books, this one really works the best!

Cleo Patra

I thought the joke in chapter seven was pretty funny.

Bernie

This really does need consideration for a pulitzer prize.

Orville Pulitzer

'The Truth About Life' Humor Books

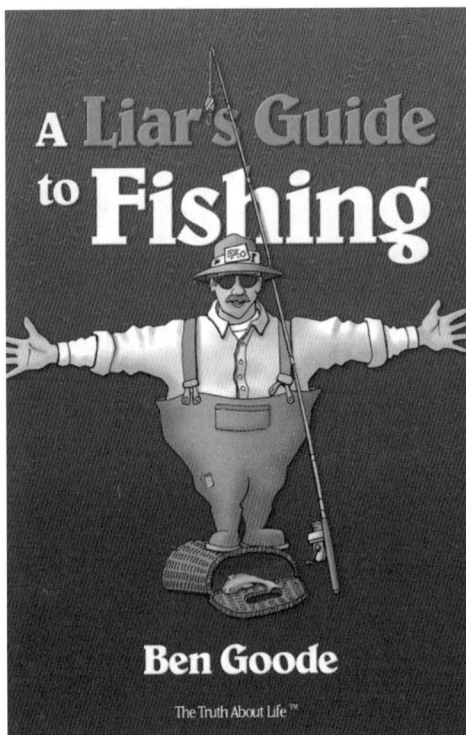

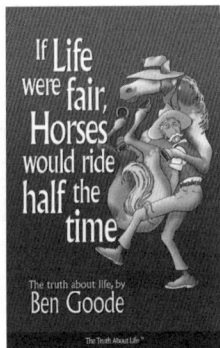

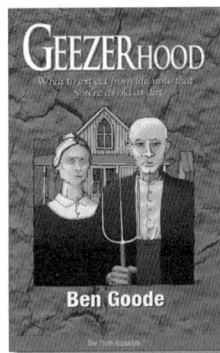

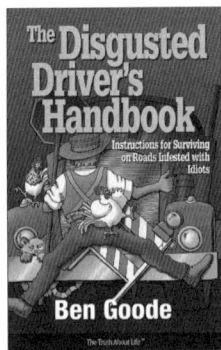

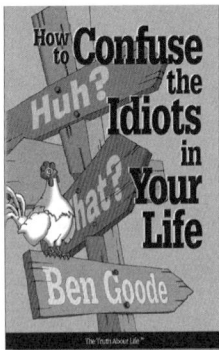

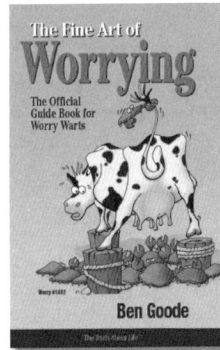

A Liar's Guide to Fishing
Ben Goode

The Truth About Life ™

If Life were fair, Horses would ride half the time
The truth about life, by
Ben Goode

The Truth About Life ™

GEEZERHOOD
What to expect from life now that you're as old as dirt
Ben Goode

The Truth About Life ™

The Disgusted Driver's Handbook
Instructions for Surviving on Roads Infested with Idiots
Ben Goode

The Truth About Life ™

How to Confuse the Idiots in Your Life
Huh?
What?
Ben Goode

The Truth About Life ™

The Fine Art of Worrying
The Official Guide Book for Worry Warts
Ben Goode

The Truth About Life ™

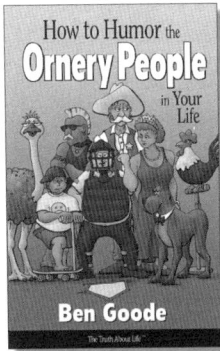

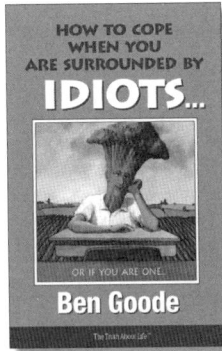

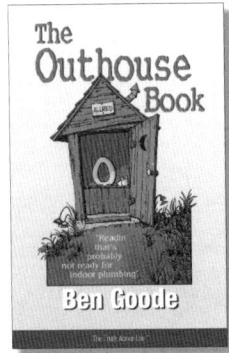

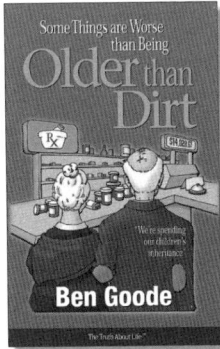

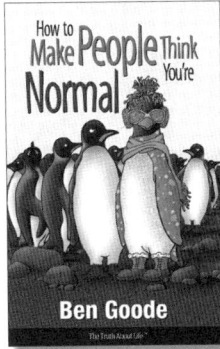

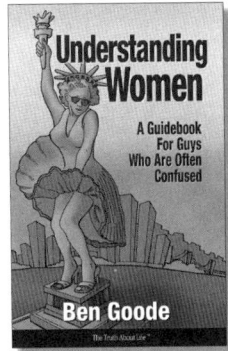

Apricot Press Order Form

Book Title	Quantity	x	Cost / Book	=	Total
_____	_____		_____		_____
_____	_____		_____		_____
_____	_____		_____		_____
_____	_____		_____		_____
_____	_____		_____		_____
_____	_____		_____		_____
_____	_____		_____		_____
_____	_____		_____		_____

All Cook Books are $9.95 US.   All other books are $6.95 US.

Do not send Cash. Mail check or money order to:
**Apricot Press   P.O. Box 1611
American Fork, Utah   84003**
Telephone 801-756-0456
Allow 3 weeks for delivery.

**Quantity discounts available.
Call us for more information.**
9 a.m. - 5 p.m. MST

Sub Total =

Shipping = $2.00

Tax 8.5% =

Total Amount
Enclosed =

Shipping Address

Name:

Street:

City: State:

Zip Code:

Telephone:

Email: